Repellents
Non-Toxic And Easy To Make Repellents To Protect Yourself From Harmful Insects

Table of Content:

Introduction

As we all know throughout the world there are millions of species of insects present and not all of them are friendly. In fact, some of them are even deadly because they carry venomous substances on their systems. However, there are some friendly insects that we knew such as butterflies and we would love to see them fly by because they are colorful and gentle.

So what we will tackle about in this book are the insects that can bring us significant harm particularly on our health and our overall wellbeing. How did I say so? An insect bite can carry diseases such as malaria, dengue, allergies, and even HIV! Mostly, mosquitoes are the carrier of the large percentage of diseases that are brought to us by insects.

I remember before when I was still a child I was really frightened because I caught an allergy that is due to an insect bite as far as I can remember it is a bite from a bug that I got out of bed.

This is the primary reason as I grow old I am always conscious about insects and I do not want them near my skin. So I did some research on how to create my own insect repellents because the repellents that can be bought on the grocery stores and pharmacies tend to have a negative effect on my skin.

Luckily, because of hard work and research, I was able to make my first all-natural insect repellent and I was very happy. Since then I had fun making different insect repellents for various insects which became my hobby, so I decided to write it on this book to impart my knowledge to you and use it for your own advantage.

The recipes are really easy to create because there are no complex ingredients that are included in the recipes so expect that you can create them easily. Let us not delay the learning anymore by starting it off immediately with the first chapter in which I will give you some background about insects so that you can understand them.

I believe that it is a crucial matter in order to repel them away from your skin. We will start now so brace yourselves from the knowledge that you will learn throughout this eBook.

Chapter 1 – The Effects of Getting Bitten By Insects

Figuring out how to hike will give you an all-out fulfillment since it gives you that feeling of testing your sturdiness and experience the fun since you will be going to visit places with good sceneries. Along these lines, this sort of activity is somewhat hazardous because this type of activity can impose you to various issues like exposing you to a wide range of bugs.

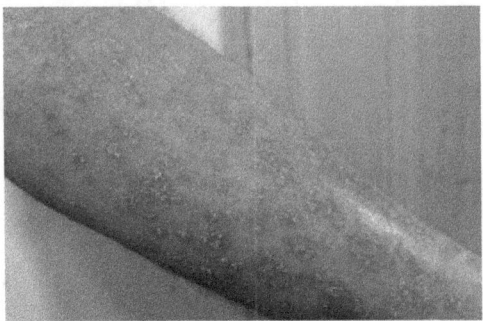

Some of them are harmless they simply love to stay nearby, while others can bring sickness that should be restored on the grounds that it can give us a destructive impact on our body

Among these creepy insects are the mosquitoes, ticks, honey bees, wasps, hornets, black flies, bugs and ants, they might be delicate in the eye, however one little bite can expedite a genuine impact our wellbeing.

By being cautious and practicing effective insect counteractive action is one of the greatest things that hikers can do to avert sickness and spreading unwanted diseases. These are the common insect-cause ailments experienced by hikers, are Malaria and Japanese Encephalitis although curable it is much better for us to prevent it rather than to cure it.

Find out About Insect Behavior

Initially, know where they colonize or residing place with the goal so that you will know where to eliminate them and where the ailments transmission happened.

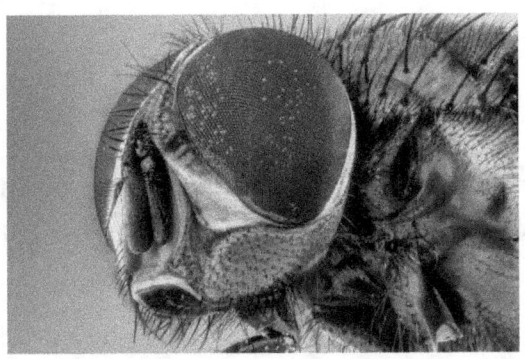

Next, find out about the insect's conduct. This will incredibly assist you with understanding whether the place that you want to travel can bring you significant exposure to those living organisms.

- What is their condition? Do they reside the inside, outside, or both?

- When would they say they are most dynamic, time? AM or PM?

- Are they present all year or do they are only seasonal?

- Do they live in urban or rustic regions?

- Are they equipped for conveying sicknesses transmitted to individuals?

Simple bite or sting?

The indications of insect bites can vary on the type of the insect and the affectability of the individual who is bitten. For instance, a few people may have little experience of irritation after they are bitten, which can go on for a minute. Others may build up an extreme resistance to it which is a good thing, however, some of us might be really affected even with one little bite which can lead to nasty swelling and even infection.

Just as insects that bite harmlessly painful or not and the worst thing is you'll encounter an insect that has venom on them.

The insects that sting include:

- ✓ *bees (bumble bees and honey bees)*
- ✓ *wasps*
- ✓ *hornets*

These stinging insects are dynamic and appear on the mid part of summer to the latter part of it when the workers search for foods to provide to their rulers that they can use for the winter season.

Here are the 2 tips that you can take advantage to know them more.

1. *Most of the time we are not noticing that we already have been bitten by insects. Since a portion of the insects that we have in the world today like the Anopheles Malaria mosquitoes don't produce sounds and don't leave an imprint in the wake of its presence.*

2. *If you were bitten by an insect which resulted in an infection, sometimes symptoms will not show up. In some cases, you may even have a mellow type of sickness and may feel that you simply have influenza or a cold, or even an undesirable skin rash.*

Hazard factors

In case you work outside or regularly participate in open air exercises, for example, outdoors or climbing, you are inclined to be at risk of insect bites. Since most of the time, the outside dress should be comfortable that is why we used to wear shorts which reveal a large segment of our skin, for example, legs and arms, that gives you a higher risk of getting bitten by insects.

When would it be advisable for me to see a medical professional?

See your doctor in the event that you have serious manifestations (for instance, in the event that you have a ton of swelling and pain) or if there is discharge, which demonstrates an infection.

Chapter 2 – Natural Mosquito Repellent Recipes

Mosquitoes are normally less dynamic toward the beginning of the day as they can't withstand the beams of the sun. Actually, they may even get got dried out and die when exposed to an excessive amount of daylight. However, it is a completely different story at night.

The minute the sun starts to set, mosquitoes start their chase for their next host, would you like to avoid them in the most ideal and regular way? Then the use of natural insect repellents will save you all the way from the irritation and illnesses that mosquito bites can bring.

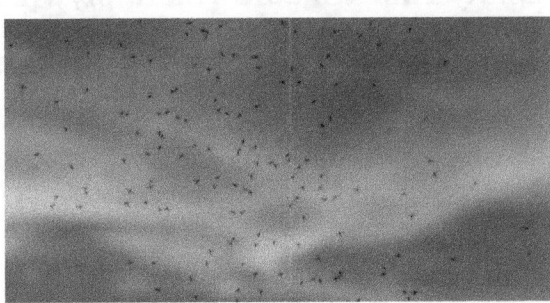

Lemon Eucalyptus Oil

Ingredients:

Lemon eucalyptus oil - 10 milliliters

Coconut or olive oil - 90 milliliters

Instructions:

1. *Get a 100 milliliters jug and pour 10 milliliters of lemon eucalyptus oil to it.*

2. *Put 90 milliliters of either coconut or olive oil to the lemon eucalyptus oil and blend them carefully.*

3. *Apply this blend generously to the affected region.*

How Many Times Should You Apply This?

Reapply this blend intermittently, particularly when you are outside.

Why this is Effective?

Lemon eucalyptus oil contains mixes like citronellal and p-methane 3,8-diol (PMD). While citronellal is accepted to demonstrate a little repellency against mosquitoes, PMD is profoundly powerful against these insects that are considered as pests.

Peppermint Oil and Coconut Oil

Ingredients:

Peppermint oil - 12 drops

Coconut oil - 30 milliliters

Instructions:

1. *Mix peppermint oil with coconut oil.*

2. *Apply this blend generously to your hands and legs.*

How Many Times You Should Do This

Execute this 2-3 times before you go outside your house.

Why This is Effective?

Peppermint oil is a kind of essential oil that functions admirably in getting rid of mosquitoes. Consolidating it with coconut oil upgrades its mosquito repellent potential and essentially makes it your own one of a kind insect repellent.

While peppermint contains mixes like limonene and menthol that keeps mosquitoes under control, coconut oil contains unsaturated fats and emulsifiers that hinder the vanishing of the anti-agents particles of peppermint oil.

Neem Oil and Coconut Oil

Ingredients

Neem oil - 9 drops

Coconut oil - 25 milliliters

Instructions:

1. *Put the neem oil to coconut oil.*

2.   *Mix well and apply this generously to the uncovered areas of your body.*

How Many Times You Should Do This?

Apply this, at any amount, two times per day.

Why This Works?

Neem oil is gotten from the seeds and products of the neem tree. It is accepted to have normal mosquito repellent properties because of its attributes and solid smell.

Truth be told, an investigation has demonstrated that 2% neem oil, when utilized in mix with coconut oil, gave huge protection guaranteed against various types of mosquitoes.

<u>Citronella Oil And Alcohol Spray</u>

Ingredients:

Liquor - 10 milliliters

Citronella oil - 10 drops

Water - 80 milliliters

Instructions:

1.   *Blend liquor and water in predetermined extents.*

2.   *Include citronella oil and blend well.*

3.   *Put this in a small container and splash on the uncovered areas of your body.*

How Many Times You Should Do This?

You should do this 2 to multiple times day by day before you head outside.

Why This Works?

Citronella oil is acquired from the leaves of the lemongrass plant. It contains numerous mixes like citronellal, geraniol, citronellol, citral, and limonene that display mosquito repellent properties.

Soda With Vinegar Mosquito Trap

Ingredients:

1 cup of vinegar

1/4 cup of soft drinks

Instructions:

1. *Get an empty jug and cut it into half.*

2. *Put the soft drink to the base part of the jug.*

3. *Take the top piece of the jug and transform it with the goal that it would look like a channel.*

4. *Place the modified portion of the container over the half of the base.*

5. *Pour vinegar into this and spot it outside your room.*

How Many Times You Should Do This

Do this at whatever point there is an expansion in the number of mosquitoes in your general vicinity.

Why This Works?

When there is the presence of soft drinks that interacts with vinegar, the response between the two discharges carbon dioxide. Carbon dioxide pulls in mosquitoes and consequently can be utilized to trap and kill them.

Chapter 3 – Bed Bug Repellent Recipes

Homemade Bug Spray

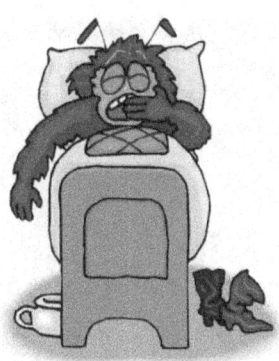

Ingredients:

Geranium essential oil – 29 drops

Citronella essential oil – 29 drops

Lemon eucalyptus essential oil – 19 drops

Lavender essential oil – 19 drops

Rosemary essential oil – 9 drops

Vodka or rubbing alcohol – 1 tablespoon

Natural witch hazel – half cup

Water or vinegar – half cup

Instructions

1. *Put the essential oils in a glass spray <u>container</u>. Include vodka or other types of alcoholic drinks and shake tremendously for it to combine well.*

2. *Add the witch hazel and shudder it to mix well.*

3. *If preferred put half teaspoon of vegetable glycerin. This is not mandatory however helps the ingredients to stay intact.*

4. *Include water and shake repeatedly. Shake every after use as the oils and water will naturally split eventually.*

How to Use

I place the container on my cabinet for easy access, and also in our first aid kit whenever I am going outdoors. I also bring with me my personally made cream for itching to protect me from bug bites.

Herbal Bug Spray

What do you need?

- ✓ Water (must be distilled)
- ✓ Rubbing alcohol
- ✓ Peppermint
- ✓ Citronella
- ✓ Catnip
- ✓ Lavender
- ✓ Spearmint
- ✓ Lemongrass

What to do?

1. Heat a cup of water and put 2-3 tbsp of herbs total in any mixture from the ingredients above. I utilize 1 tbsp each of spearmint, citronella, and lemongrass, and also put in some cloves preferably the dry ones.
2. Combine carefully, coat and let the heat subside.

3. *Remove the water from the herbs and put it in a cup of witch hazel or rubbing alcohol.*

4. *Pour in a spray container in a humid area. It is advisable to keep it in the fridge for maximal preservation.*

5. *Use as necessary.*

Essential oils

Thyme, lemongrass, lavender, and tea tree oils can be utilized to diminish bed bugs for good. Basically blend five to ten drops of these with water, empty it into a spray container and splash on the surfaces that are necessary to be sprayed.

It can both repulse and slaughter bed bugs as a result of its normal properties. It can likewise be utilized on the body as an anti-agents, yet the centralization of the essential oils ought to be almost no for that utilization.

Rubbing Alcohol

In the event that you tapped the connection above about the potential for causing a flame with hand-crafted insect repellent, at that point you will realize that rubbing alcohol was somewhat in charge of the blast. That doesn't need to stop you, be that as it may, from using this personally made solution.

The motivation behind why the general population in that news report had their home burst into flames is on the grounds that they were utilizing alcohol close to open fire, so simply recall that significant wellbeing tip on an instance that you choose to utilize this technique. Try not to utilize alcohol on close flame or notwithstanding consuming incense.

Chapter 4 – Lice Repellent Recipes

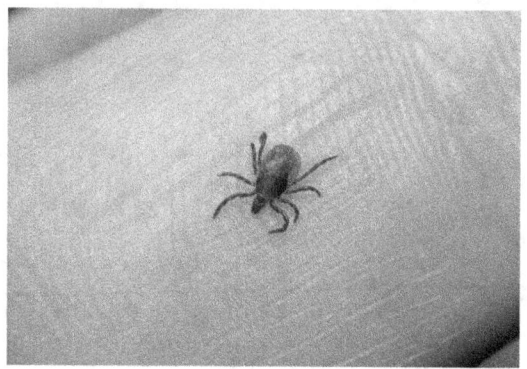

Recipe #1

Blend the accompanying essential oils in a 3 ounces spray container, filled most of the way with water. In case that you have a much larger container, modify the essential oil sum as needs be.

What do you need?

- ✓ *Tea tree oil - 9 drops*
- ✓ *Lavender oil - 4 drops*
- ✓ *Rosemary oil - 4 drops*
- ✓ *Peppermint oil - 4 drops*

Shake a long time before you use it and rest assured that those nasty lice will be off the hook!

Recipe #2

- ✓ *Water - 5 oz.*

- ✓ *Vodka - 5 oz.*

- ✓ *Essential oils - 79 drops*

- ✓ *Neem oil - 2 teaspoons*

- Blend the majority of the oils in an 8 ounces spray container.

- Shake the container and spray on hair every morning, and again when going to places where lice presentation is likely!

As a model, for my last shower, I add more oils, and after that increased the alcohol content to help diminish them.

I combined the accompanying: 2 teaspoons of neem oil a couple of squirts of argan oil, 29 drops tea tree essential oil, 19 drops eucalyptus essential oil, 19 drops lavender, 5 drops cinnamon leaf oil, 4 drops geranium oil.

At that point filled the container with more vodka, alongside a dash of refined water, and shook it to consolidate everything really well. In the event that you are utilizing for youngsters under 10, you can supplant the eucalyptus oil with an alternative oil on the rundown, or a blend of oils.

Recipe #3

What do you need?

- ✓ *Water - 2 oz.*

- ✓ *Tea tree oil - 11 drops*

- ✓ *Spray container – this sort of plastic container is likely a decent alternative too.*

✓ *Lavender oil - 5 drops (either Hungarian or Bulgarian)*

Technique

- Mix the above ingredients in the spray container and splash on hair.

- No compelling reason to rinse it out.

- To Prevent Lice: Spray on hair day by day toward the beginning of the day or potentially around evening time. Work through the whole head of hair.

- To Remove Lice: Spray on the hair around evening time and search over hosed hair with absolute attention to detail toward the beginning of the day.

<u>Quick Notes:</u> Hungarian Lavender has a sweet aroma, and Bulgarian Lavender has an increasingly herbaceous fragrance. So pick depending on your preference.

Neem Oil Shampoo

Neem oil, similar to tea tree oil, is likewise viewed as a common insect spray. Numerous botanists use it to diminish bugs in their nurseries. It is successful yet it has a dreadful smell.

Add a couple of teaspoons to your ordinary cleanser (plain cleanser, not molding) or some unscented fluid Castile cleanser to make a neem oil cleanser.

Apple Cider Vinegar

Is there anything apple juice vinegar isn't useful for? On an instance that there is, I don't think I've discovered it. When you cleanse, wash your hair with apple juice vinegar. Or then again simply douse your hair with ACV, let it sit for a couple of minutes and after that brush out your hair with a nit brush.

Essential Oil Treatment

- ✓ *Sesame seed oil - 1/4 cup*

- ✓ *Neem oil - 1/8 cup*

- ✓ *Tea tree basic oil - 11 drops*

- ✓ *Eucalyptus oil - 6 drops*

- ✓ *Rosemary basic oil - 4 drops*

- ✓ *Lavender essential oil - 9 drops*

Soak hair with apple juice vinegar and apply the oil blend to your hair.

Spread it with a shower top and leave it in for 6 or 8 hours (think about it in the event that you don't have time amid the day).

Search over with a nit brush the following morning and cleanser as you ordinarily would. Utilize this treatment consistently for the multi-week basis to dispose of head lice.

Epsom Salt and Water

When you mix it with water may get dried out and diminish lice. To utilize, apply 2-3 tablespoons Epsom salt broke down in 1/4 container warm water (or more if necessary) to the scalp/hair.

Enable the solution to sit until the hair is completely dry, at that point wash before beginning with Step 1.

Coconut Or Olive Oil and Essential Oils

As referenced above, in this investigation, a cream that included 10% tea tree and 1% lavender oil was 97.6% powerful in disposing of lice, while bug sprays like pyrethrins and piperonyl butoxide were just 25% successful.

Chapter 5 – Additional Insect Repellent Recipes

Vodka Surprise – Spray On

To start with, blend everything aside from the essential oils. When the base is in, include the oils and shake well for quick use!

What do you need?

- ✓ Witch hazel - 3 tbsp.

- ✓ Almond oil, jojoba oil, or avocado oil. - 3 tbsp.

- ✓ Vodka - half tsp.

- ✓ Lemon eucalyptus essential oil - 54 drops

- ✓ Lavender oil essential oil - 16 drops

- ✓ Cedarwood essential oil - 14 drops

- ✓ Rosemary essential oil - 14 drops

- ✓ Spray container - 9 ounces

Skin Smoothing – Spray On

Essentially combine the majority of the ingredients, shake, and shower! The skin relieving benefits originate from both witch hazel and apple juice vinegar. Numerous sorts of toner and other great items to help prevent skin break out, perspiring, razor consumes, and the sky is the limit from there!

What do you need?

- ✓ *Apple juice vinegar - half cup*
- ✓ *Witch hazel - half cup*
- ✓ *Eucalyptus - 39 drops*
- ✓ *Spray container - 9 ounces*

Non-Edible Alcohol – Spray On

Include the majority of the essential oils into a spray container, and afterward include liquor and shake. After these ingredients consolidate, put in the witch hazel and give it another great shake!

What do you need?

- ✓ *Rubbing alcohol - 1 tablespoon*

- ✓ *Witch hazel - half cup*

- ✓ *Glycerin - 1 teaspoon*

- ✓ *Water or vinegar - half cup*

- ✓ *Geranium essential oil - 29 drops*

- ✓ *Citronella essential oil - 29 drops*

- ✓ *Lavender essential oil - 19 drops*

- ✓ *Lemon eucalyptus essential oil – 21 drops*

- ✓ *Rosemary essential oil - 9 drops*

- ✓ *Spray bottle - 9 ounces*

Simple Essentials Homemade Insect Repellent – Rub On

What do you need?

- ✓ *Transporter oil of your preference (avocado oil, grapeseed oil, coconut oil) - 2 tablespoon*

✓   *The essential oil of your choice - 20 drops*

✓   *Spray container*

Add the transporter oil to your container, and afterward blend in the essential oils. Shake before you rub this oil blend onto your skin!

Water-based Combination Insect Repellent – Spray-on

What do you need?

✓ *Lemon juice - 3-4 tablespoons*

✓ *Lavender essential oil - 14 drops*

✓ *Vanilla concentrate - 3-4 tablespoon*

✓ *Distilled water*

Consolidate all the ingredients in your preferred spray container, and shake.

In the event that you would prefer not to buy refined water, just bubble water for a similar impact.

The Easiest Essential Oil Recipe – Rub On or Spray On

What do you need?

- ✓ *Lemon eucalyptus essential oil*

- ✓ *Choose either one of the following: Witch hazel, sunflower oil, neem oil, and almond oil.*

Blend 1 part of the essential oil with 11 drops of the witch hazel or oil. To blend it up, have a go at utilizing more than one kind of oil!

Smell Like a Mosquito Repelling Candle – Rub On

What do you need?

- ✓ *Citronella essential oil - 11 drops*

- ✓ *Eucalyptus essential oil - 11 drops*

- ✓ *Cedar fundamental oil - 5 drops*

- ✓ *Your preferred oil (jojoba, neem, and fennel) - 4 tablespoons*

Bugs Hate Mouthwash – Spray On

What do you need?

- ✓ *A mouthwash of your choice*

- ✓ *1 spray container*

Just shower mouthwash on yourself as a simple personally-made insect repellent. Always remember despite that it is a mouthwash you should not drink it because we already transformed it into an insect repellent, just be cautious with that to prevent any unwanted incidents that might happen.

Zest Cabinet Raid – Spray On

What do you need?

- ✓ *Water - 1 cup*

- ✓ *Witch hazel or rubbing alcohol - 1 cup*

- ✓ *Dried herbs any of the following: peppermint, lavender, catnip, or spearmint - 4 tablespoons*

- ✓ *Dried cloves - 2 pieces*

- ✓ *Spray container*

Consolidate the water, herbs, and cloves then heat to the point of boiling. When it is already heated, fill the container, blend, spread, and let the solution cool totally. At the point when the mix is cool, strain the herbs and throw them away.

Keep the water and include the rest of the ingredients, witch hazel or rubbing alcohol. Store this handcrafted creepy crawly repellent in a cool spot like the icebox.

Castile Soap Soup – Spray On

What do you need?

- ✓ *Fluid Castile cleanser - 9 teaspoon*

- ✓ *Neem oil - 1 teaspoon*

- ✓ *Refined water - 4 containers*

- ✓ *Spray bottle - 1 piece*

Consolidate all the ingredients, shake, and apply!

The Marinator – Spray On

The marinator is known for the smelliest handcrafted bug repellent formula that is around for a long time. In any case, as it dries the smell disperses to people. To ticks and mosquitoes, this stuff keeps directly on smelling and annoying for them resulting in a total diminishing of them!

What do you need?

- ✓ *Dried sage - 2 tablespoons*

- ✓ Thyme - 2 tablespoons

- ✓ Mint - 2 tablespoons

- ✓ Rosemary - 2 tablespoons

- ✓ Lavender - 2 tablespoons

- ✓ Apple juice vinegar - 32 ounces

- ✓ Spray bottles

Blend all the ingredients in the glass container. Seal well, and put it in a place you won't neglect to shake day by day. Shake well each day for 2-3 weeks.

After this tincture has had sufficient energy to marinate, strain the herbs and keep everything in the fridge. Since this stuff is so incredible, blend a balance of the blend and water in the splash bottles.

Peppermint and Vanilla Tincture – Spray On

What do you need?

- ✓ Vodka - 1 container

- ✓ *Vanilla concentrate - 1 tablespoon*
- ✓ *Cloves - 1 tablespoon*
- ✓ *Peppermint extricate - 1 tablespoon*
- ✓ *Spray bottle*

Consolidate everything into the container, shake, and let it sit for a while. This custom made bug repellent works better the more it is permitted to sit as long as a month. In case you go this course, try to shake day by day. Note: you may need to strain out the cloves in the wake of soaking.

The Italian Job – Spray On

What do you need?

- ✓ *Refined water - half container*
- ✓ *Vodka - half container*
- ✓ *Cleaved crisp basil - 1 container*
- ✓ *spray bottle - 1 piece*

Convey water to a moving bubble, and include the basil. Heat this blend to the point of boiling, spread, and let sit for at least 6 hours.

At the point when time is up, strain out the herbs and empty the fragrant water into the shower bottle. Include vodka, shake, and your natively constructed bug repellent is prepared to go!

Vanilla Extract – Spray On or Rub On

The vanilla concentrate can be added to any of the plans of the trivial oil for included security. Moreover, it can really be utilized without anyone else to repulse mosquitoes.

Rub it on the skin, or blend it with a balance of witch hazel and water for a brisk, tyke well disposed, and shower capable form. It is also known that vanilla is great for the skin because it has properties that nourish and brings suppleness to our skin.

So you are hitting to birds in one stone, you are protecting yourself from the harmful effects of insect bites and at the same time enhance your appearance.

Do not hesitate now and try this recipe out and you will surely know what I am talking about. This is probably the best for you if you are looking to have a good lotion and insect repellent in an all-in-one action.

Conclusion

Wow, that was a great learning experience for all of us. We had able to learn the different insect repellents to keep us safe at all times. Aside from that upon bringing those recipes to life you will gain a lot of benefits from it such as you will not get any side-effects because the ingredients are all natural.

The good thing with the recipes that we discussed is that you will save a lot of money as well from buying ready-made insect repellents in the market minus the artificial ingredients that can impose a significant risk in our health in the form of cancers, allergies, and many more than you can ever imagine.

One suggestion that I can give you is after you have created the certain insect repellent recipe from this book, try a small portion first on your skin before applying it generously. This will help you see if the recipe is compatible with your skin.

I am not saying that because the recipes are all-natural you will not take any precautionary measures at all, it is always better to be safe at all times.

Although some of the recipes that I have included here obviously does not smell well because its primary purpose is to repel those unwanted insects away from you. However, you can also blend the recipes with the essential oils of your choice to make them smell more pleasing.

As far as I can remember I have experimented some and found significant success on it. The good thing is the recipes smelled better and at the same time did not lose their effectiveness in chasing away insects.

Since then those recipes became a part of my daily routine right now I am really happy that I have the confidence that I and my family are safe from the harmful effects of insect bites.

As you have read in this book a while ago the different recipes that you can use to repel different kinds of insects and as a beginner, you will notice that the recipes that I have included are composed of the user-friendly ones and the more complex recipes.

My advice starts first with the simple recipes from there you will have the chance to get a glimpse of how to blend properly. So once you mastered blending you can level up by creating the much more complex recipes and practice it very often so that the next time that you will be doing it you will become more comfortable.

That's it! I hope you enjoyed this book and I suggest that you refer this book to your friends after you read it because it is always a good decision to become protected from insect bites. As the world evolves, a new strain of diseases that is transferrable through a bite of an insect is truly frightening. The pieces of knowledge that you have found here are truly priceless. Why? Because you cannot put a price on the health of you and your family.

www.ingramcontent.com/pod-product-compliance
Lightning Source LLC
Chambersburg PA
CBHW070448290526
45791CB00005B/2097